Where Should Mom Live?

Living Arrangements for Older Adults

Laura Town and Karen Hoffman

Omega Press

Zionsville, IN 46077

ISBN: 978-0-9969832-5-9

Production Credits:
Authors: Laura Town and Karen Hoffman
Publisher: Omega Press
Photos: All images used under license from Shutterstock.com

Social media connections:
Laura Town
Twitter: @laurawtown
LinkedIn: https://www.linkedin.com/in/lauratown

Karen Hoffman
LinkedIn: www.linkedin.com/pub/karen-kassel/62/2b/915/

CONTENTS

WHERE SHOULD MOM LIVE?
Living Arrangements for Older Adults

Older adults account for a substantial and growing portion of the population. More than 47 million people aged 65 and older lived in the United States in 2015, accounting for nearly 15 percent of the total population. That number is expected to rise dramatically through 2030, with estimates suggesting that 74 million Americans—roughly 21 percent of the population—will fall into this group. This increase is due to the aging of the Baby Boom generation (individuals born between 1946 and 1964).

Today's older adults have a longer life expectancy than their parents' generation, but they still face many health-related challenges associated with age. Chronic health conditions such as heart disease, diabetes, and cancer are widespread among older adults. Dementia and Alzheimer's disease are also prevalent. The number of individuals affected by these conditions has increased over time and is expected to continue increasing in the future. Health conditions, as well as general age-related physical changes, may lead to difficulties with mobility, vision, hearing, and cognition. These difficulties often manifest in struggles with basic self-care and home care tasks like bathing, doing laundry, and cooking. Tasks such as these are often referred to as activities of daily living (ADL).

Income is also a concern for many older individuals, especially women and members of minority population

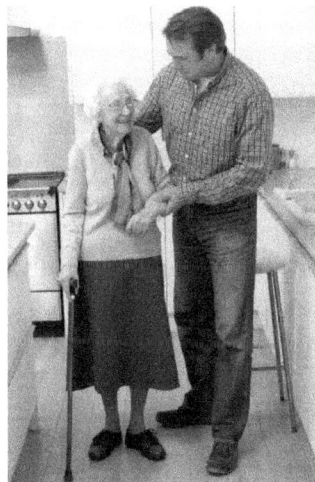

Credit: Monkey Business Images

groups. In addition, continued aging strains financial assets, and individuals 75 and older tend to be less secure than those between the ages of 65 and 75. Nutrition and healthcare may suffer when older adults face economic problems, as may the ability to secure adequate housing.

What all of this means is that caring for an aging loved one will be part of the future for many of us. One aspect of providing that care is assessing your loved one's living arrangements and changing those arrangements over time. Most older adults want to live independently for as long as possible. As health, economic, and family situations change, your loved one's needs and wishes may also change.

Finding the living arrangement that works best for your loved one, you, and your family is very important. Every situation is different, so while living with a caregiver may work well for one family, an assisted living facility may be the best solution for another. To make an informed decision, you should know the facts concerning each type of living arrangement.

Stay at Home

Most of us would prefer to live in our homes unaided until our death. While this is not possible for many older adults, your loved one will probably choose to stay at home as long they can. In the beginning, this will not involve a lot of planning or changes around the house, but as time progresses, changes will need to be made for both convenience and safety. Additional help may be needed around the house for daily cleaning tasks, laundry, maintenance, or companionship. When working with your loved one to make changes around the house or to their daily routine, try to ensure that these changes will not negatively impact their sense of independence. This can be difficult to balance, but preserving as much of their independence as possible will likely make a huge difference to your loved one.

Preserving Independence

Helping your loved one preserve their independence is important because it can help increase and preserve mental acuity in older adults. You might feel compelled to take control of everything the moment your loved one experiences age-related struggles because you think this will help relieve some of their burden or stress. In fact, the exact opposite is likely to happen. As mental and physical aspects of the aging process manifest, your loved one will begin to realize that soon they may be unable to do many of the things they once enjoyed. This realization will turn any loss of independence, no matter how small, into a sign of what is to come in the future. The following checklist discusses tips for helping your loved one maintain independence while they still live at home.

Checklist: Helping preserve independence at home

☐ Stock the refrigerator and pantries with easy-to-make foods, such as sandwich materials or meals that can be made in the microwave. If your loved one has experienced problems using the microwave, consider posting directions for microwave use nearby.

☐ If your loved one enjoys cooking, offer to help them cook a few meals each week, but make sure not to take over. Allow your loved one to do as much of the preparation as possible, only lending support when necessary.

☐ If your loved one can no longer cook and you are not able to help, arrange with Meals on Wheels to deliver hot meals to your loved one.

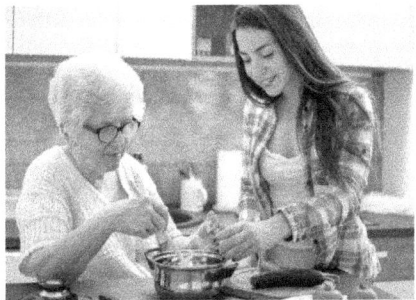
Credit: Bojan Milinkov

☐ Help your loved one set up automatic bill payments for their monthly bills.

☐ For bills that cannot be set up through bill pay (snow removal, local newspaper delivery, landscaping, etc.), suggest that your loved one create a calendar with dates for when these payments need to be made. Once the check is delivered, your loved one can check it off on the calendar.

- ☐ Help your loved one set up daily routines to make the management of daily tasks easier and less stressful.

- ☐ If your loved one is used to doing the grocery shopping, help them create a grocery list so the trip is easier.

- ☐ If your loved one tends to become tired or overwhelmed at the grocery store, offer to go along. Be there for support and companionship, but do not interfere unless they need or ask for your help. Alternately, you could help your loved one create an online shopping list and have the groceries delivered to their home.

- ☐ Buy an electric tea kettle so that your loved one can make tea or instant coffee without having to worry about using the stove. Make sure you purchase a device with an automatic shut-off feature.

- ☐ Be observant about tasks that are going undone in your loved one's home (e.g., cleaning, laundry, grocery shopping) and offer to help. Your loved one may be resistant to asking for help with everyday tasks, but if you offer, they may be less hesitant to accept.

- ☐ If your loved one has trouble with incontinence, place incontinence pads close to the toilet for your loved one to use.

- ☐ Avoid taking control. Your loved one can still do many things on their own, so only offer help when needed.

- ☐ If your loved one used to enjoy going for walks (or other similar activities) but has stopped due to a fear becoming lost or fatigued, offer to go for a walk with them on a set day or two each week.

Meals on Wheels and Other Meal Services

Meals on Wheels America is a senior nutrition program that works to ensure no elder adult goes without food. Approximately one million meals per day are provided by Meals on Wheels in the United States, with delivery typically occurring around lunchtime. These meals are served at senior centers or can be delivered straight to a person's home. If your loved one has limited independence and does not cook anymore (either for safety reasons or because they do not want to), signing them up for Meals on Wheels could be a good solution. The checklist below discusses some of the aspects of this program.

Checklist: Basics about the Meals on Wheels program

- ☐ The individual receiving meals must be homebound (not able to leave the home, or it is difficult to leave the home) and at least 60 years old.

- ☐ Those under 60 can also receive meals if they have a disability or their income is low enough to meet the requirements. These requirements differ by state and program, so check with your local organization to see if your loved one qualifies.

- ☐ You can sign a loved one up to have meals delivered to their house; individuals do not have to sign themselves up for the program.

- ☐ Prices per meal are generally set on a sliding scale but can be anywhere from free to $8 per meal.

- ☐ Some areas offer meal packages where you can pay for meals by the week or month.

- ☐ You will need to fill out an application (or answer questions over the phone) regarding any dietary restrictions your loved one has. In some areas, you may also be required to provide a referral letter from a doctor or social worker.

- ☐ Meals on Wheels programs employ nutritionists, so meals are healthy and well balanced. All meals satisfy 1/3 of an individual's daily recommended nutrition and include grains, protein, and vegetables; milk, bread, and fruit or dessert are also often provided.

- ☐ Some programs will also provide pet food at a discounted rate once a month for seniors who have pets living with them.

- In some states (Pennsylvania, Maryland, Florida, and others), Meals on Wheels programs offer grocery shopping services to homebound seniors. Sometimes $5–$10 is charged for this service in addition to the cost of groceries.

- For individuals who have meals delivered weekly, non-perishable food items are delivered in advance of very bad weather. This way, if a volunteer cannot make it to your loved one's home because of the weather, food is still available.

- Meals are generally served only on weekdays (Monday–Friday), but frozen meals can be provided for the weekends if needed.

- Once you sign your loved one up, meal delivery can generally start within a day or two. It may take longer in some areas, but they try to start as soon as possible. In areas with the greatest need for this service, there may be a waiting list.

- Meals on Wheels has programs across the country in both rural and urban areas. You can visit their website to find a provider near you. Additional contact information for this program can be found in the Resources at the end of the book.

Other meal or grocery delivery services are available and may be appropriate for your loved one. The majority of these services are privately owned and cater to individuals and families at all ages and stages of life. These services are generally more expensive than Meals on Wheels and are not specifically designed to meet the nutritional requirements of older adults. The food delivered usually requires preparation, rather than being ready-to-eat. These services do offer the advantage of greater flexibility in terms of food choices. They may also deliver essential non-food items, like toothpaste, soap, and shampoo.

Meal delivery services typically bring all of the ingredients required to make a meal to your loved one's door, though some services bring pre-made meals that just require reheating. Ingredients are typically accompanied by recipes for preparing the food. Meals are ordered online from the service's website or mobile application and require about a week for delivery. One delivery typically contains ingredients for three nights' worth of meals. Cost is $12 per person or less per meal and some services charge a membership fee. Shipping fees vary by service, with some offering free shipping.

Blue Apron is an example of a meal delivery service. It does not charge a membership fee, but you must create an account in order to use the service. Once the account is created, meal kits are automatically delivered each week and the credit card on file is charged. Two-person and family meal plans are available. Depending upon the plan selected, two to four meals per week may be ordered from that week's meal options. Blue Apron was one of the first services of its kind in the United States, but many options are currently available, including HelloFresh, Plated, and Chef'd.

Grocery delivery services allow you or your loved one to go online through a website or mobile application, select the needed products, and place an order. Orders are generally delivered the same day, often within a matter of hours. Users pay the cost of the groceries purchased plus additional fees for the service. Fees vary by company. Some companies require a paid membership while others charge per-order fees. Delivery fees may also apply and may be dependent upon the cost of the groceries and the retailer from which they are purchased.

Shipt is an example of a grocery delivery service with a membership fee, which may be paid annually or monthly. Once your order is placed through the website or app, a Shipt shopper goes to the store of your choice and purchases the requested items. If the shopper has questions about the order, they will contact you or your loved one via text message for clarification. Prices paid for individual items reflect a slight markup over the store price to help cover the costs of shopping for and packing the order. Orders under $35 are charged a delivery fee, while orders over $35 are not. Other grocery delivery services include Instacart, AmazonFresh, and Peapod. Many grocery stores are starting to offer shopping services as well, though some retailers require that groceries be picked up in-store rather than being delivered.

Home Modifications

In order for your loved one to safely stay in their home, you may need to make several modifications. These changes are made not only for your loved one's safety but also to increase their independence and overall well-being. Changes to the house can be expensive, but they are necessary and can prevent greater expenses later on. Some changes that should be made for safety include modifications to prevent falling, tripping, and burns. If your loved one is experiencing dementia or other cognitive issues, locking up medications and hazardous products and making modifications to prevent wandering may also be necessary. The following checklist details some changes that can be made to the home.

Checklist: Home modifications for safety

- ☐ Remove excess clutter from the house.

- ☐ Ensure that stairways are well lit; this could include adding light switches at the top and bottom of each stairwell.

- ☐ Add reflective and/or colorful tape to the edge of stairs to increase visibility.

- ☐ Install extra lighting in all rooms.

- ☐ Replace flip-style switches with rocker switches, which are easier to turn on and off.

- ☐ Install securely anchored handrails in stairwells, bathrooms, and long hallways. Consider installing rails on both sides of stairwells.

- ☐ Secure or remove throw rugs and other tripping hazards.

- ☐ Add adhesive safety strips to tub or shower floors.

- ☐ Install grab bars and seats in showers.

- ☐ Install an elevated toilet or purchase a raised toilet seat.

- ☐ Install ramps for small sets of stairs (one or two steps) if your loved one struggles with steps. For longer flights, install a chair lift.

- Remove raised door thresholds when possible. If thresholds cannot be removed, no-step rubber threshold ramps can be purchased.

- Widen doorways to accommodate mobility aids (wheelchairs, walkers) when possible. If doors cannot be widened, swing-clear hinges can be installed.

- Provide low-level storage in the kitchen and other areas of the house to lessen the need for reaching and climbing.

- Increase space between furniture to ensure ample clearance; this may mean removing some pieces of furniture.

- Replace doorknobs and round faucet handles with easy-to-turn lever handles.

- Purchase a digital voice reminder device for the door your loved one uses to exit the house. The reminders will sound when the door opens; a voice recording will instruct your loved one to turn off the lights and remember the house keys, or whatever messages you program into the device.

Home Services

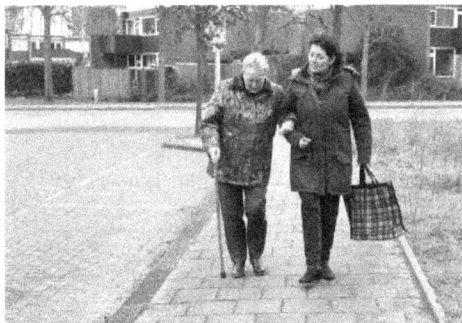

Credit: Nancy Beijersbergen

While your loved one is living at home, you may find it beneficial to look into home service options. Your loved one may not need medical services or help with personal care unless they have a preexisting medical condition, but they may benefit from companion services or homemaker services. Companion services can be arranged for once a week or multiple times a week, as needed. If your loved one is living with their spouse or another family member, then perhaps they only need someone to come in once or twice a week. Homemaker services provide help with cooking, cleaning, laundry, food shopping, and other similar tasks. Even if your loved one is independent enough to live at home, both of these services can be helpful to decrease loneliness and frustration. If your loved one has always done the cooking and cleaning but is no longer able to perform these tasks all the time, they may become easily frustrated if they are unable to successfully complete these things alone. To find local home service providers in your area, consult the Resources at the end of the book. The checklist below discusses the duties performed by different home service providers.

Checklist: Types of duties performed by home services

Homemaker Services:

- ☐ Cooking
- ☐ Washing dishes
- ☐ Laundry
- ☐ Changing bed sheets
- ☐ Dusting
- ☐ Vacuuming
- ☐ Cleaning bathrooms
- ☐ Taking out trash
- ☐ Organization
- ☐ Medicine schedule reminders
- ☐ Pet care
- ☐ Houseplant care
- ☐ Errand assistance
- ☐ Grocery shopping

Companion Services:

- ☐ Conversation

- Recreational activities (games, movies, walks, favorite hobbies, puzzles, etc.)
- Transportation to doctor's appointments or the grocery store
- Assistance in running errands
- Cognitive stimulation
- Help with phone calls
- Help with email or letter writing
- Light cleaning and cooking

Personal Care Services:

- Assistance with bathing
- Assistance with dressing
- Assistance with toileting
- Feeding assistance and monitoring
- Medicine reminders and monitoring
- Cooking
- Cleaning
- Laundry
- Changing bed sheets
- Shopping
- Providing transportation to appointments or the grocery store

Everybody experiences aging differently, and every older adult is unique in their daily wants, needs, and struggles. Therefore, there are no specific guidelines for when your loved one may need or want different types of home services. In addition, some older adults may be hesitant to seek or ask for assistance around the home. The following checklist describes some indicators that your loved one may be in need of additional help around the house.

Checklist: *When should my loved one start receiving home services?*

☐ The laundry is piling up without being washed.

☐ You notice that your loved one wears clothes repeatedly without laundering them.

☐ Your loved one has not changed the bed sheets in weeks.

☐ Your loved one has started sleeping on the couch because the bed sheets and/or blankets need to be washed.

☐ The sink is always full of dirty dishes.

☐ The refrigerator has an abundance of old and/or spoiled food.

☐ The cabinets and pantry contain mostly old or expired food.

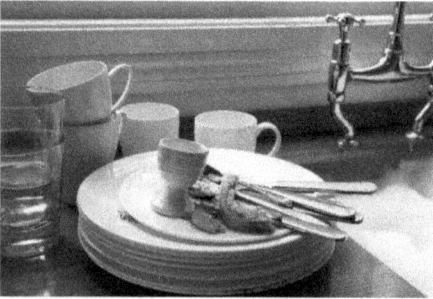
Credit: sirtravelalot

☐ There is very little food in the house because your loved one has not gone grocery shopping.

☐ Your loved has been going without eating because they do not want to cook.

☐ Your loved one has a pet whose food dish is empty most times when you visit.

☐ Your loved one has difficulty bathing and/or dressing and is resistant to asking you or another family member for help.

☐ You notice that your loved one has bruises or injuries from falling when getting into or out of the shower or bathtub.

☐ Extra medication is present in your loved one's pill organizer because they have forgotten to take their pills multiple times.

- [ ] Unopened letters and correspondence pile up around the house.

- [ ] Your loved one's house has fallen well below the level of cleanliness your loved one has typically maintained.

- [ ] A layer of dust is present on tables, bookshelves, and other stationary items.

- [ ] Newspapers and other recyclables have started piling up.

- [ ] The carpet appears to not have been vacuumed in weeks, if not longer.

- [ ] The floors are covered with mud, dirt, and debris from a lack of sweeping and mopping.

- [ ] You realize that your loved one has very little social interaction and spends most days only watching television.

- [ ] The only person your loved one talks to most weeks is you.

- [ ] Your loved one frequently complains about feeling lonely.

- [ ] Your loved one is no longer able to drive but has various appointments during the day.

You do not need to arrange companion and homemaker services through an agency or outside source. A relative, family member, friend, or neighbor could stop by a few times a week to visit your loved one and help around the house. If you or your loved one has a large support network close by, such as friends, relatives, church companions, and/or community members, you can create a Caring Bridge website to set up a schedule of what everyone can do to help. (Please see the Resources for more information.) However, a large support group is not always available, so you also have the option to hire someone to perform these tasks. Both independent employees and caregiver service organizations are available; you can also sometimes find help through local churches, colleges with social work and nursing majors, senior centers, and community aid agencies. Before hiring someone for these positions, you should go through a thorough interview process. Consider the following checklist of questions to ask during an interview.

Checklist: Questions to ask when hiring companion and homemaker services

- [ ] What is their previous work experience?

- [ ] If your loved one has a medical condition, have they worked with someone with that condition before?

- [ ] Will they submit to a background check?

- [ ] Do they have references?

- [ ] Have they ever been fired from a home service position before? If so, what was the reason for termination?

- [ ] In order to ensure they get along well with your loved one, are they willing to be hired on a trial basis first?

- [ ] Would your loved one prefer someone of the same gender to provide care, especially if they will be helping with bathing or dressing?

- [ ] Do they seem responsible? Have they answered all phone calls and/or emails in a timely manner? Did they show up to the interview on time?

- [ ] Do they have an agreeable personality/attitude?

- [ ] Do they appear to be patient?

- [ ] If they are interviewing to be a companion, what activities do they plan to do?

- [ ] Can they adjust their cooking style to meet the dietary needs of your loved one?

- [ ] Are they CPR and/or first aid certified?

- [ ] If they are applying for a position in which they will be driving your loved one, how is their driving record?

- [ ] Do they have a reliable form of transportation? Do they have car insurance?

- [ ] If they are applying for a position where they will be expected to clean, are there any tasks they will not do? For example, are they opposed to cleaning toilets or washing dishes by hand?

Home Healthcare

As your loved one's age advances, or if medical conditions occur or worsen, you may need to consider home healthcare services. Home healthcare could also be beneficial to your loved one if they have difficulty taking medications properly. Home healthcare services are generally provided by a nurse or physician's assistant and can help with administering medications, bathing, eating, and sometimes even physical therapy. Home healthcare can be provided in your loved one's home as often as they need the services. The aide can visit weekly, daily, or even provide 24-hour-a-day care. If your loved one has a condition that requires 24-hour care, hiring an around-the-clock care provider will

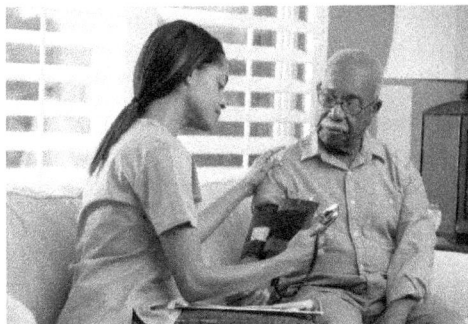
Credit: Monkey Business Images

generally allow them to stay in their home longer, avoiding the need to change their living arrangements.

Checklist: When to hire home healthcare

☐ Your loved one needs help with medications.

☐ Your loved one needs wound care.

☐ Your loved one is experiencing medical problems beyond your abilities (e.g., diabetes, heart disease, or blood clots).

☐ Your loved one needs daily or weekly injections.

☐ Your loved one gets infections easily.

☐ Your loved one requires specialized medical equipment.

☐ You are making frequent visits to the doctor for things that could be handled by a nurse at your loved one's home.

- ☐ Your loved one has particular diet and nutritional needs.

- ☐ Your loved one needs help bathing and dressing.

- ☐ Your loved one requires physical therapy.

Before hiring someone to work with your loved one, you should do some research into the company or service you are considering. Some resources to help with this research are included at the end of the book. The following checklist discusses what to look for when hiring home healthcare.

Checklist: What to look for when hiring home healthcare

- ☐ Does the healthcare service run background checks on their employees?

- ☐ Are the employees trained to care for patients with your loved one's specific medical condition?

- ☐ What kind of training do the employees receive?

- ☐ What skill level are the employees? RNs? CNAs?

- ☐ How are the employees monitored to ensure a high quality of care?

- ☐ What policies are in place to handle problems if they arise?

- ☐ Will you be able to personally choose/interview the employees who will be working with your loved one?

- ☐ Can the home healthcare worker take your loved one to the hospital if necessary, or will an ambulance need to be called?

- ☐ Will the home healthcare worker wait with your loved one until you get to the hospital?

- ☐ Will you need to provide meals for the home healthcare worker, or will they bring their own?

- ☐ Is it possible to do a trial day/week to see how the employee and your loved one interact together?

- Will your loved one be assigned a regular healthcare worker or will the person change each week/day?

- If a regular healthcare worker is not available to come due to illness or other factors, will a replacement be sent?

- How will you be notified of the replacement?

- How long has the company been in business?

- What kind of reputation do they have within the community?

- Is the service only available during the week, or do they have weekend care as well?

- Is the company an approved Medicare or Medicaid provider?

- Does the company honor the Patient's Bill of Rights (the patient's overall rights in terms of care, such as being treated with respect)?

- Will the company provide you with a sample plan of care for a client with your loved one's condition?

- What is the company's policy on patient confidentiality?

- Are fees fixed or do they work on a sliding scale?

- Is there financial assistance available when needed?

- Is the company licensed by the state?

- Do the company's representatives seem friendly and helpful?

- Does the company have relationships with dietitians, counselors, and/or other specialists? Can they provide referrals if/when they are needed?

- How quickly do services begin?

Geriatric Care Manager

When you feel it is time to hire home services, consider finding a geriatric care manager who will oversee your loved one's home care. Geriatric care managers are generally trained in social work, counseling, nursing, or other professions related to the field of geriatrics (a branch of medicine specializing in the care of older adults). The role of a geriatric care manager is to aid families and their loved ones with the many challenges associated with finding appropriate care. A care manager gets to know your loved one as well as your family and then works to suggest the best care in terms of insurance, resources, and the reputation of the service provider, if applicable. These managers help facilitate care, whether in the home or in a residential facility. If, as a caregiver, you are overwhelmed by determining the best living arrangements for your loved one, or you are unsure if your loved one's current living arrangements are in their best interest, you may want to consider a geriatric care manager.

Geriatric care managers are rarely, if ever, covered by insurance companies or Medicare, and their fees may prohibit you from considering this option. However, sometimes a sliding scale fee can be arranged depending on the company or individual being hired. If you are interested in this type of service, conduct research to find an agency that provides the services you want at the best price. The checklists below discuss the services that most geriatric care managers offer, signs to help you determine which services might be of use to you, and what to look for in a care manager.

Checklist: What services do geriatric care managers provide?

- ☐ Customize all services and suggestions specifically to your loved one's needs by performing in-depth interviews with caregivers, family, and your loved one.

- ☐ Recommend a care plan tailored to your loved one's needs.

- ☐ Set up and attend doctor's appointments with your loved one.

- ☐ Ensure communication between doctors and your loved one and family.

- ☐ Act as an advocate for you and your loved one in cases where there are disagreements with a living facility, hospital, or doctor.

- ☐ Manage your loved one's medication schedule.

- Help plan for the future needs of your loved one based on their current health and prognosis.

- Help avoid preventable or unnecessary hospitalization, incorrect placements, and/or duplicated services.

- Suggest the most appropriate forms of home care services.

- Recommend and facilitate social and recreational activities.

- Monitor your loved one's condition and suggest changes in housing arrangements and/or services when necessary.

- Help select living arrangements and organize all details to facilitate the move.

- Help ensure smooth transitions between living situations.

- Provide crisis intervention and counseling, as needed.

- Recommend legal assistance by working with elder care attorneys.

- Facilitate management of finances by working closely with the individual your loved one has given power of attorney.

- Monitor your loved one's well-being, watching for signs of emotional, physical, and/or financial abuse.

- Alert family and caregivers to any problems.

Checklist: Signs you might need a geriatric care manager

- Your loved one has no family members nearby and you are trying to manage care from another state.

- The environment your loved one is currently living in is unsafe, but you do not know how to fix the situation.

- You and/or your family are unsure what care decisions would be best.

- You have been trying to research living arrangements, medical needs, and other care-related elements for your loved one, but you are confused and frustrated.

- You are having difficulty communicating your loved one's needs to the home healthcare service providers they are currently using or the facility where they are currently living.

- Your relationship with your loved one's current service providers or the facility where your loved one is currently living has become hostile and/or increasingly strained.

- Your family disagrees about the best course of action regarding care decisions and living arrangements.

- You and/or your loved one have many questions regarding financial and legal matters.

- Your loved one is in need of a strong care advocate.

Checklist: *What to look for when hiring a geriatric care manager*

Geriatric Care Management Company:

- How long has the company been providing this service?

- What kind of training do they receive?

- Will the company provide references for the care manager?

- Do all employees undergo a background check?

- What types of backgrounds do their geriatric care managers have (e.g., social work, nursing, or counseling)?

- How does the company supervise their care managers?

- How often will you be updated about your loved one's situation?

- How much do they charge for a consultation?

- How much do they charge for services?

- Do they offer sliding scale fees?

- Do they offer the services you need most?

- Can they show you an example of a care plan they have used for a client with your loved one's specific medical condition or issues?
- Are care managers available on weekends and holidays?

Independent Geriatric Care Managers:

- How long has the individual been offering geriatric care management services?
- How many clients has the individual worked with to date?
- What kind of training has the individual had?
- Will the individual submit to a background check?
- Will the individual provide a list of references?
- What is the person's background (e.g., nursing, social work, or counseling)?
- Is the individual a certified geriatric care manager?
- Is the person familiar with the area in which your loved one lives and the resources available in that area?
- How often will you be updated on your loved one's care?
- How much does the individual charge for services?
- How many other clients will the person have in addition to your loved one? Or will your loved one be the person's primary client?
- Is the individual friendly and approachable?
- Do you like the person? Do you think you could trust and work with this person long term?
- Does the individual seem responsible? Has the person answered your phone calls and/or emails in a timely manner?
- Can the individual provide examples of care plans that he or she has drawn up for other clients?
- Does the person offer the services you need most?

- ☐ Is the person in contact with an elder care attorney? Or does the person have a strong knowledge of elder care laws?

- ☐ Is the individual available for emergencies?

- ☐ Does the person provide consultation on weekends and holidays, if necessary?

- ☐ Does the person belong to any professional organizations in their field?

Leaving Home

When caring for your aging loved one, a time may come when you notice them experiencing greater difficulties remaining independent. You may become concerned about the safety of their home environment, and you may find it difficult to relax or sleep through the night because of these concerns. These are signs that you should reassess your loved one's living situation. The following checklist highlights some signs that, either individually or in combination, could point to it no longer being safe for your loved one to live alone.

Checklist: Signs it is no longer safe for your loved one to live alone

- ☐ Your loved one has presented fire safety concerns, such as trying to cook but leaving the stove on or ignoring the smoke detectors.

- ☐ Your loved one gets confused or scared easily in their own house.

- ☐ Your loved one needs someone around 24 hours a day.

- ☐ Your loved one is afraid to be alone.

- ☐ Your loved one is having difficulty successfully bathing or dressing.

- ☐ Your loved one has had a few minor falls and/or a more severe fall that caused injuries.

- ☐ Your loved one is becoming increasingly withdrawn and/or depressed.

- ☐ Weight loss has become apparent because your loved is not eating regularly.

- ☐ Your loved one's ability to communicate has begun to decline.

- ☐ Your loved one's is having obvious hygiene difficulties, such as not bathing, forgetting to brush teeth or hair, and wearing the same clothes each day.

- ☐ Your loved one is not taking medication properly.

- ☐ You feel that your loved one would not know what to do in case of an emergency, an illness, or an injury.

Move in with Caregiver

One option to consider when your loved one is no longer able to live alone is for them to move in with a caregiver or to have a caregiver move into your loved one's home. Caregivers are usually children or close relatives of the older adult. If you choose this option and become your loved one's caregiver, you need to consider home healthcare services, adult day care, routine changes, and safety concerns. If your loved one has a serious medical condition, their needs in these areas may be pronounced.

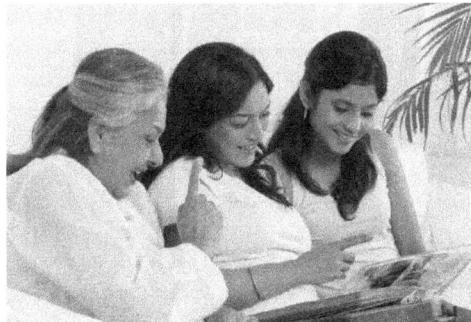

Credit: India Picture

When your loved one must leave their home, you have several options. The first one many people consider is having their loved one move in with them. This is not the correct option for everyone, but for some it works well. You need to find the option that works best for you and your family. Consider the checklists below to determine if having your loved one move in with you is a good option.

Checklist: Should my loved one move in with me?

- [ ] Can my loved one safely live alone (see *Checklist: Signs it is no longer safe for your loved one to live alone*)?

- [ ] Do I have extra room in my house for my loved one?

- [ ] Do I have the monetary resources to hire someone to be with my loved one during the day if necessary, or will my schedule allow me to be home when needed?

- [ ] Is this option more affordable than a live-in facility?

- [ ] Can I handle the emotional stress this may cause?

- [ ] Can my children/spouse handle the emotional stress?

- [ ] Will my job situation allow for me to leave at a moment's notice to take care of any emergencies that may arise while my loved one lives at home?

- [ ] Have my loved one and I decided together that this should be the next step before considering an independent or full-time living facility?

- [ ] Do I have relief care options in place to avoid becoming burned out?

- [ ] Do I want full control over the care my loved one receives?

- [ ] Would I feel safer if my loved one was not living at home alone?

- [ ] Do my loved one and I get along well with one another? If you and your loved one do not communicate well in low-stress situations, then it is likely that having them move in with you will create unnecessary stress for both of you.

- [ ] Can I be patient with my loved one when they get frustrated or have a bad day?

- [ ] Can my home be easily (and affordably) converted to meet the physical needs of my loved one?

☐ Does my loved one need around-the-clock, skilled medical attention?

Checklist: Pros and cons of moving in with a caregiver

Pros:

☐ It is less expensive than a residential facility.

☐ Your loved one is close by.

☐ Your loved one will be in a familiar environment.

☐ You will be able to easily spend more time with your loved one.

☐ You will have more control over the type of care your loved one receives.

☐ You will be more involved with your loved one's care.

☐ You can ensure your loved one is getting daily exercise and cognitive stimulation.

☐ You will be able to monitor for fraud and scams more easily.

Cons:

☐ Caregivers have a high chance of burnout.

☐ Caring for an individual with serious health issues can be extremely stressful.

☐ Being a primary caregiver is time consuming.

☐ Your sleeping, eating, and daily habits may have to change to accommodate your loved one's habits.

☐ Your daily routines could be disrupted, particularly if you have young children.

☐ You will be responsible for your loved one's safety and well-being.

☐ Your loved one may eventually have to be moved to a residential facility if their health or abilities decline.

☐ You may need to hire home healthcare services if your loved one has a progressive medical condition.

Before deciding to have your loved one move in with you and your family, you should know the duties and responsibilities you will have. Live-in caregivers to individuals with chronic, progressive medical conditions may become burned out because they do not understand the amount of work, and sometimes stress, that comes with this role. As an example, consider Alzheimer's disease. In the United States in 2017, more than 16 million caregivers provided roughly 18.4 billion hours of care to individuals with Alzheimer's disease. That is a great deal of unpaid work, and it is often done in addition to regular full- or part-time employment. Taking on the role of live-in caregiver is a momentous decision. The following checklist discusses some of the responsibilities you will have if your loved one moves into your home.

Checklist: What are the roles of a live-in caregiver?

☐ Implement a daily routine.

☐ Plan nutritious, healthy meals.

☐ Prepare medications and monitor if they are taken correctly.

☐ Watch for signs of adverse reactions to medications.

☐ Organize daily physical activities and exercise, if possible.

☐ Organize daily activities to engage the mind.

☐ Ensure your loved one has opportunities for socializing.

☐ Plan various activities to keep your loved one from sitting around most of the day.

☐ Organize your loved one's participation in spiritual activities, if this is something they have always done or they want to do.

☐ Plan visits with friends and family.

☐ Prevent your loved one from experiencing too much stress.

☐ Assist your loved one with bathing, dressing, and toileting when needed.

- ☐ Help your loved one with daily grooming (shaving, brushing teeth) when needed.

- ☐ Stay patient and calm when helping your loved one.

- ☐ Work to ensure your loved one's safety in the home, as well as out in public.

- ☐ Assess and modify the house for safety as needed.

- ☐ Ensure that your loved one is getting enough sleep.

- ☐ Arrange doctor and specialist appointments.

- ☐ Arrange and/or provide transportation to appointments and outings.

- ☐ Act as an advocate for your loved one with doctors, and potentially other family members. (This is primarily the responsibility of a healthcare agent.)

- ☐ Manage, or help manage, your loved one's finances. (This is primarily the responsibility of a durable power of attorney for finances.)

- ☐ Hire home services (home healthcare, homemaker, and/or companion services) when needed.

If you have made the decision to have your loved one move in with you, this will likely be a difficult time for your loved one. They will be leaving their home, which will greatly decrease their independence. Moving in with an adult child or relative on top of that may seem to your loved one as though they are no longer trusted or able to provide their own care. Maintaining independence is important when your loved one moves in with you, because increased independence can be beneficial to their overall well-being. The following checklist discusses some tips for helping your loved one maintain their independence after the move.

Checklist: Tips for maintaining independence when living with a caregiver

☐ Encourage your loved one to help around the house with small tasks such as setting the table, washing dishes, folding laundry, etc.

☐ Have your loved one help you prepare meals, especially meals they used to cook regularly.

☐ Ask your loved one to help with the baking, if that is something they enjoy.

☐ Ask for their opinion on cooking; maybe have them taste the food and offer suggestions.

☐ Try not to do everything for your loved one. They can still help out in many ways.

☐ If your loved one is having difficulty performing a particular task, offer to help but do not take over or do the task for them.

☐ Make sure to give your loved one choices about food and chores.

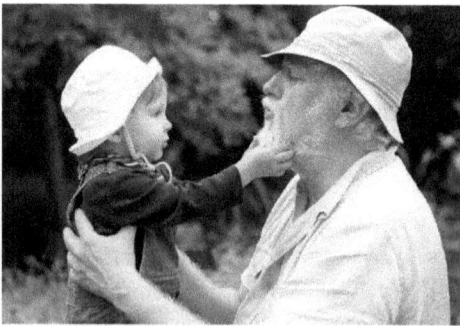

Credit: Ana Blazic Pavlovic

☐ If you have young children, encourage your loved one to help care for them. Spending time with kids can be a low-stress situation for people who are experiencing physical or cognitive problems, because they are less likely to feel as though they are being judged. It could also help bring back good memories of your loved one's childhood.

- Ask your loved one to help care for your pet (if you have one). Your loved one could help take the pet for walks or help feed the animal. Pets can be very therapeutic.

- Encourage your loved one to help you with gardening or taking care of indoor plants, if that is something they enjoy. Always stay with your loved when using tools in the garden that could lead to injury.

- Plan outings once a week if your loved one is able, and give them a choice of the location.

- If your loved one has stopped participating in hobbies or activities because their health has made it difficult, offer to participate in those activities together. For example, you could go for walks together or work on a craft they enjoy.

- If your loved is having incontinence problems, do not make a big deal out of it. Buy disposable underwear and leave them in the bathroom your loved one uses; tell your loved one where you placed the underwear, but do not mention it again unless necessary.

- Engage your loved one in decisions about their health, activities, and options whenever possible.

Caregiver Agreements

If your loved one is unable to remain independent and provide their own care, a family member may step in to become a caregiver. Sometimes, the caregiver goes to your loved one's home for several hours each day to provide care. In other situations, the caregiver may move in with your loved one or your loved one may move in with the caregiver, as discussed earlier. This can create both a financial and emotional hardship for the caregiver, especially if the caregiver must give up a steady job with benefits to provide care. If one individual is providing the majority of care for your loved one, your family may want to create a caregiver agreement that allows your loved one to pay the caregiver for the care they provide. The following checklists provide basic information about caregiver agreements as well as information that should be included in the caregiver agreement. For a sample care agreement, see the Resources.

Checklist: Basics about a caregiver agreement

- ☐ A caregiver agreement is a contract between an ill individual and a caregiver to list caregiving responsibilities and compensation for care provided.

- ☐ A caregiver agreement can also be called a personal care agreement, long-term care personal support services agreement, elder care contract, family care contract, or caregiver contract.

- ☐ A caregiver agreement can be used to compensate a family member who has made a great personal sacrifice in order to provide care for a loved one. This prevents the caregiver from experiencing undue financial hardships due to their caregiving responsibilities.

- ☐ The caregiver agreement should be put in writing. This allows the caregiver and family members to have a record of the caregiver's responsibilities and compensation as well as provide proof to Medicaid and other government assistance programs that the transfer of money between your loved one and the caregiver was for caregiving services and not a gift.

- ☐ A caregiving agreement can help avoid family conflicts over who should provide care and what type of care they should provide.

- ☐ Because a caregiving agreement may affect the inheritance, all family members should help construct the caregiving agreement, especially the amount the caregiver will be compensated.

- ☐ A caregiver agreement is used to stipulate payment for future caregiving services. It should not provide compensation for past caregiving services.

- ☐ A caregiver agreement provides your loved one with peace of mind that they will be cared for if they are no longer able to provide their own care.

□ A lawyer is not needed to complete the caregiver agreement, but it may be beneficial to consult a lawyer for complicated agreements.

Checklist: Characteristics of a caregiver

□ Often an adult child of the older adult, although adult grandchildren, other relatives, or friends may also provide care

□ Should live close to your loved one

□ Should be someone your loved one knows, not a stranger

□ Often has few personal responsibilities, such as no minor children living at home

□ Is willing to give up a paying job if necessary to care for your loved one, provided they will be paid for providing care to your loved one

□ Willing to take on the time commitment and responsibility needed to care for a loved one

□ Responsible and even-tempered

□ Understands the list of responsibilities as well as how to perform the needed tasks

Checklist: Information to include in a caregiver agreement

□ The date care should begin. For individuals with progressive medical conditions, this may be a vague date in the future based on the progression of the disease.

□ How long the agreement is in effect (e.g., one year, five years, for the lifetime of the individual).

□ A detailed description of care to be provided. You may want to have a care assessment conducted in the home or consult your loved one's medical records to help determine the care needed. Specifically defining the care tasks to be completed and the time they will take will help compensation and time expectations be more reasonable. See *Checklist: Types of caregiver duties listed in a caregiver agreement* for more information.

☐ Provisions for expanded care responsibilities as your loved one's disease progresses or their health deteriorates.

☐ Where the care will take place (e.g., at the loved one's home, in the caregiver's home). Allow for a change of location as needed based on your loved one's needs.

☐ How many hours of caregiving will be provided each week. Depending upon your loved one's needs or medical condition, the number of caregiving hours may need to be given on a sliding scale. Language should allow for flexibility, such as "up to 20 hours per week" or "no less than 160 hours per month."

☐ The amount of compensation for the caregiver. Compensation for care should be similar to what the family would pay a third party to provide care. The family may need to do some research into the amount they would pay a caregiving service for a similar level of care. The amount of compensation should reflect the complexity of caregiving duties and the time spent on caregiving duties.

☐ When the caregiver will be compensated (e.g., weekly, bi-weekly, monthly).

☐ Provisions for raises in the future to compensate for a job well done.

☐ Provisions for living expense compensation (e.g., room and board, utilities) if your loved one lives with the caregiver; also make sure that homeowners insurance covers liabilities such as work injuries.

☐ Provisions for health insurance and other benefits for the caregiver, especially if they resigned from a job with benefits to provide care for your loved one.

☐ Your loved one's responsibility vs. the caregiver's responsibility for paying withholding taxes and Social Security.

- Provisions for incidental out-of-pocket expenses, including but not limited to home modifications for safety.

- Determine who will write the checks. This should be the power of attorney for finances; if the caregiver is the power of attorney, consult a trustee or other legal representative.

- If the caregiver will be responsible for transportation, stipulate the level of car insurance that is needed.

- Provisions for respite time or vacation time for the caregiver.

- Provisions for caregiving backup if the caregiver goes on vacation, gets sick, or needs respite time.

- A statement that the agreement can be modified only by mutual agreement by both parties. Any modifications should be put in writing and signed and dated by both parties.

- A statement that the caregiver can void the contract if the caregiving duties exceed their abilities. For example, a caregiver may feel unqualified to care for your loved one in the late stages of Alzheimer's disease.

- Signatures of both parties and the date. If your loved one is not legally competent to sign the document, their durable power of attorney for finances or conservator can sign for them. If the caregiver and your loved one's legal financial representative are the same person, consider consulting an attorney.

Checklist: Types of caregiver duties listed in a caregiver agreement

- Hygiene care (e.g., bathing, dressing, grooming)

- Nutrition (e.g., cooking, special diet considerations, feeding, grocery shopping)

- Mobility (e.g., assisting with transfers from the bed to a chair)

- Monitoring medications

- Tracking changes in health

- ☐ Companionship

- ☐ Monitoring for safety (e.g., driving, home safety, medication safety)

- ☐ Housekeeping (e.g., cleaning, laundry, dishes, errands); may list individual tasks if needed

- ☐ Outdoor maintenance (e.g., mowing lawn, trimming bushes, raking leaves, snow removal)

- ☐ Finances (e.g., paying household bills, paying medical bills, balancing the checkbook); note that this may be the duty of a power of attorney rather than the caregiver

- ☐ Car maintenance (e.g., taking your loved one's car to the shop for oil changes)

- ☐ Transportation to appointments and events; consider mileage in compensation

- ☐ Consulting with physicians and other medical personnel; note that this may be the duty of a healthcare agent rather than the caregiver

- ☐ Creating a daily log of activities; this will help with Medicare or other documentation as well as provide evidence of services provided

- ☐ Recording payment of expenses for government assistance documentation

Caregiver Burnout

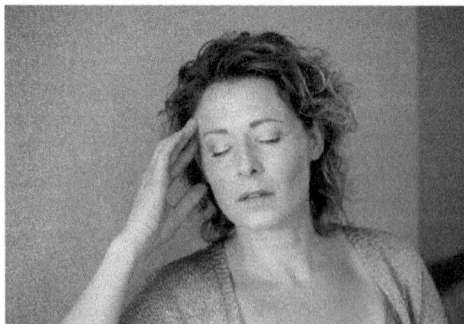

Credit: mimagephotography

If you are the primary caregiver for a loved one with a chronic medical condition, you may suffer the effects of caregiver burnout over time. Caregiver burnout occurs due to an accumulation of stress and responsibility that the caregiver experiences. If your loved one moves in with you, a routine will likely develop. However, as your loved one's condition progresses, this routine will probably become more complicated, which will ultimately leave you with more responsibility and less time for yourself. The signs of caregiver burnout are gradual, but you need to watch for them in order to avoid later complications. Being aware of the signs will also enable you to work toward reversing the effects. The following checklist discusses the signs of caregiver burnout.

Checklist: Signs of caregiver burnout

- ☐ You feel more overwhelmed than usual.

- ☐ You do not exercise or relax because you feel that there is no time.

- ☐ Your anxiety levels have started increasing.

- ☐ You have lost your temper with a loved one because they are not responding the way you want or expect.

- ☐ You are yelling at and/or becoming angry with coworkers, loved ones, and friends for no reason.

- ☐ Your emotions change quickly and drastically (e.g., you are angry one minute and extremely sad the next).

- ☐ You are not sleeping well due to stress or anxiety.

- ☐ You find that you are exhausted all the time.

- ☐ You are frequently giving up social and family events.

- ☐ You have not spent time with friends or participated in enjoyable activities in months.

- ☐ You no longer enjoy activities you once favored.

- ☐ You feel that you are unable to give your loved one the help they need.

- ☐ Your weight or appetite has changed.

- ☐ You have been ill more often than usual.

- ☐ You are having trouble concentrating on tasks.

- You are having difficulty remembering appointments or events.

- You have had thoughts of suicide.

- You have had thoughts about hurting your loved one.

- You find yourself wishing it would all be over so that your stress could end.

If you think you might be suffering from caregiver burnout, seek help for yourself and assistance with your caregiving responsibilities. Numerous support groups exist where you can meet with other people in your area who are experiencing similar difficulties. If you need a break from caregiver duties, consider taking a short vacation or having family members or a service come in one or two afternoons a week to give you time for yourself. The checklist below discusses some options for services that could help give you a break from your caregiver duties.

Checklist: Respite care and adult day care

Respite Care:

- Respite care provides you with a few hours to get out of the house and have some time to yourself.

- It occurs in your home, so your loved one would not have to leave.

- It gives your loved one a chance to interact with another person.

- It can offer you extra time to do errands.

- It helps prevent caregiver burnout.

- Friends, family, or neighbors can provide respite care.

- Community organizations offer respite care services.

- You can hire services such as homemaker and companion services to provide respite care (see Home Services).

☐ Some residential facilities offer short-term stays for respite care (one night to a few weeks).

Adult Day Care:

☐ Adult day care is a place where your loved one is cared for by trained staff while you are at work, running errands, or taking a needed break.

☐ You will be able to relax knowing that your loved one is safe and cared for.

☐ Transportation is sometimes provided to and from the day care facility.

☐ Adult day care is offered in a location outside of your home.

☐ Most centers are open between seven and ten hours a day.

☐ Some facilities have weekend and evening hours.

☐ Most centers have social workers and nurses on staff.

☐ Some adult day care centers specialize in providing care for specific medical conditions, such as Alzheimer's disease.

☐ These facilities supply nutritious meals and snacks throughout the day.

☐ Assistance taking medication is provided.

☐ Your loved one will engage in light physical exercise.

☐ Physical, occupational, and speech therapy are generally offered at these facilities.

☐ These facilities often teach relaxation techniques.

☐ Many facilities offer pet therapy and music therapy.

☐ Your loved one will be provided with activities to stimulate their mind.

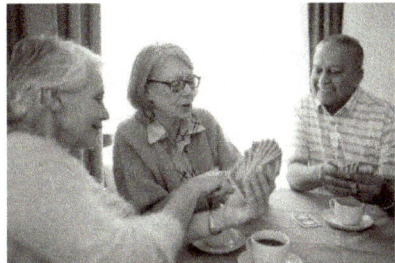

Credit: wavebreakmedia

- ☐ Your loved one will be able to interact with others and engage in social activities.

- ☐ Activities such as games, gardening, field trips, and crafts are planned throughout the day to keep your loved one entertained and active.

- ☐ Some facilities offer counseling for both your loved one and your family, if needed.

- ☐ Medicaid generally covers most, if not all, adult day care costs.

- ☐ Private insurance and long-term care insurance will sometimes cover the cost of adult day care.

Move to Assisted Living

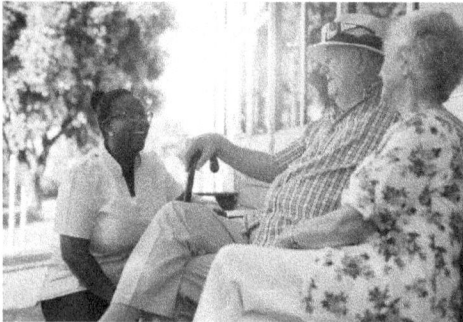

Credit: Jacob Lund

If you decide that having your loved one move in with you is not a good decision for you and your family, consider an independent care facility. Independent care facilities are also referred to as assisted living facilities, adult living centers, and supported care facilities. These residences allow those living there to have a greater sense of independence than they would experience in a hospital or nursing home while providing assistance with day-to-day activities.

Moving your loved one to an independent care facility or an assisted living facility can be a tough decision. You would generally take this step either when your loved one can no longer live alone or when your loved one's needs are too great for their primary caregiver to meet. Independent facilities do not offer around-the-clock skilled medical care. If this is needed, then you should consider a nursing home or other full-time care facility. The following checklist details some signs that your loved one, or you as their caregiver, might want to consider moving your loved one to an independent living facility.

Checklist: *Signs an independent living facility could be beneficial*

Your Loved One:

- ☐ Has started showing signs of disorientation or confusion.
- ☐ Has become lost while walking or driving in familiar areas.
- ☐ Has recently become more isolated, even depressed at times.
- ☐ Experiences little to no socialization during the day.
- ☐ Falls often.
- ☐ Has experienced difficulty cooking.
- ☐ Often neglects to eat or take medications.
- ☐ Is not safe in their current living environment due to increased physical or mental deficits or symptoms of chronic medical conditions; however, the person can still perform activities of daily living independently or with minimal help.

The Caregiver:

- ☐ Has begun losing sleep due to worrying about a loved one.
- ☐ Experiences extreme anger, sadness, and/or aggression because of stress and/or caregiver duties.
- ☐ Loses patience with their loved one often.
- ☐ Consistently gives up social or work events.
- ☐ Does not have time alone to rest and recuperate.
- ☐ Loses or gains weight due to stress.
- ☐ Experiences health problems.
- ☐ Has begun drinking alcohol, using drugs, or smoking to deal with stress.
- ☐ Can no longer keep up with their caregiver duties.

- Cannot physically help their loved one up if the individual falls.

- Has begun to resent their loved one for their physical limitations or medical conditions.

The services that independent living facilities provide depend on the individual facility. Some facilities specialize in particular types of care, such as memory care for individuals with Alzheimer's disease or other forms of dementia. However, the following checklist highlights some of the services these facilities often provide.

Checklist: Services independent facilities often provide

- Housing, either individual apartments, suites, or shared rooms

- Housekeeping services

- Laundry services

- Three meals per day, often provided in a group setting; however, most facilities will allow residents to dine alone in their rooms if they want to

- Assistance with eating, such as if food needs to be cut into smaller pieces

- 24-hour staff for assistance with any needs that may arise

- Recreational activities and events

- Therapeutic activities, such as music therapy and pet therapy

- Activities to help promote exercise.

- Relaxation activities such as meditation and yoga

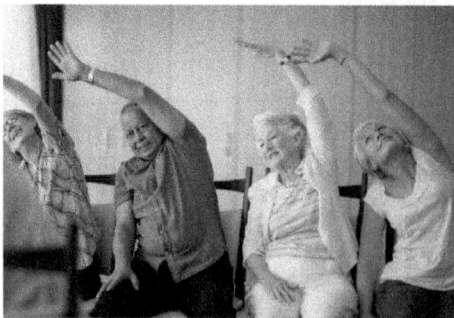
Credit: wavebreakmedia

- ☐ Assistance with bathing, dressing, and toileting as needed

- ☐ Assistance with medications, including both reminding residents when to take medications and what dose of medication to take

- ☐ 24-hour monitoring of the facility

- ☐ Emergency call systems in all rooms

- ☐ 24-hour security around the facility

- ☐ Counseling and therapy services

- ☐ Physical and speech therapy

- ☐ Transportation to doctor's appointments

- ☐ Barber and beautician services for residents

- ☐ Limited health services

- ☐ Consultations from a nutritionist when needed

- ☐ Frequent visits from a nurse on staff to ensure the resident is doing well

Before choosing an independent facility, you and your loved one, if possible, should visit the place multiple times to get a feel for the atmosphere. You should also do research into the services that facility offers as well as their individual policies. Consider the following checklist of what to look for in an independent care facility.

Checklist: Questions to consider when looking for an independent living facility

- ☐ Do they have a special unit/facility geared toward your loved one's specific medical condition?

- ☐ What behaviors will result in a resident being asked to leave?

- ☐ Will residents who experience physical and cognitive declines due to age or medical conditions need to move out, or does the facility have the ability to care for them?

- ☐ Do they offer hospice services if needed? Or will the person need to be transferred to a nursing home?

- ☐ Do residents have single apartments or will they share with others?

- ☐ How many residents are normally in a living area together?

- ☐ What is the ratio of staff to residents?

- ☐ How often do nurses check on residents?

- ☐ Do they accept residents in wheelchairs?

- ☐ Do they accept residents with oxygen tanks?

- ☐ Are there options for prepared food if residents decide they do not want to cook?

- ☐ Are the grounds and rooms of the facility maintained well? Or are they run down and dirty?

- ☐ What are the outdoor areas of the facility like? Is the facility by a busy street? Are there safe pathways for walking?

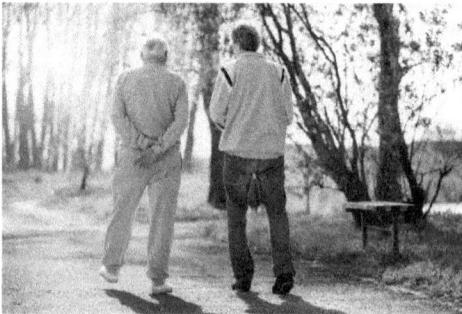

Credit: adriaticfoto

- ☐ Does the staff seem friendly when you visit?

- ☐ Are employees outgoing?

- ☐ Do the other residents at the facility appear to be happy?

- ☐ Can you visit your loved one at any time? Or are there visiting hours?

- ☐ Do they provide outings for the residents to local stores or attractions? If so, how often do these outings happen?

- ☐ What is the supervision like on the outings? If your loved one gets separated from the group, will there be enough staff to notice your loved one is missing?

- Does the facility accept your loved one's insurance plan?

- What extra costs are included at the facility that are not generally covered by insurance? For example, some activities or programs are not covered by insurance.

- Does the facility have any citations against them currently?

- Has the facility had any citations in the past? If so, how serious were the citations and how long ago did they occur?

- What is the facility's policy regarding medication? Do they hand out medication daily to residents? Or are residents expected to keep their own medications?

- What is the facility's policy in the case of a medical emergency?

- Does each apartment have an emergency response system to easily call for help?

- What is the staff coverage/assistance like on the weekends and holidays?

Independent living facilities are generally reserved for those who do not need skilled medical care but may require assistance in their day-to-day activities. As such, these facilities would be more appropriate if your loved one is experiencing minor physical or cognitive deficits or minor complications associated with a medical condition. If they experience greater functional decline or disease-related issues worsen, you will likely need to move them from an independent care facility to a full-time care facility. For example, when my dad was in the earlier stages of Alzheimer's disease, he was in an assisted living facility. All went well for five or six months. Then one day I received a call from the facility. Dad had hit someone. This was the first fight Dad was ever in. Completely unprovoked, Dad started punching people. After evaluation at a

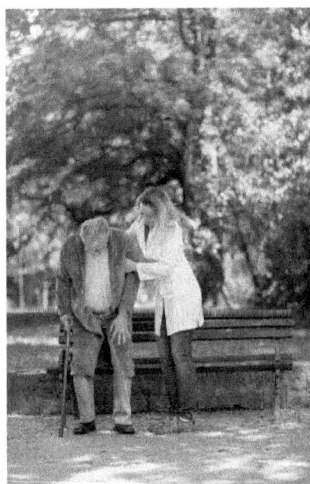

Credit: Lucky Business

43

psychiatric facility, he was cleared to return to assisted living. Shortly after that, he hit someone else and returned back the psychiatric facility for additional assessment. In my state, an individual patient who has three psychiatric stays can be denied entrance by any nursing home. Dad was at two. It was very clear at this point that I had to move him to a full-time care facility quickly if I wanted to have some choice in where he was staying.

Move to Full-Time Care Facility

Full-time care facilities are generally either nursing homes or settings very similar to nursing homes that specialize in caring for older adults with significant physical declines, cognitive declines, or disease-related problems. If your loved one requires medical attention, 24-hour care, assistance with walking and dressing, and/or around-the-clock supervision, a full-time care facility could be helpful. These facilities employ teams of nurses, social workers, therapists, nutritionists, and doctors to assist residents with their day-to-day needs. In addition, most nursing homes have common areas where activities are held as well as options for communal dining so that residents can socialize with one another if they choose to.

After Dad's aggressive episodes at the assisted living facility, I knew I had to decide which full-time care facility I wanted to place him in. Dad was already on the waiting lists for the best nursing homes, but no spots were open. A nursing home with a "below average" rating was close to my home, so close that it was within walking distance. I talked to the geriatric psychiatrist and agonized over what to do. He reminded me that I had to do what was best for both my father and myself. I placed dad in the nursing home, and I wasn't happy about it. However, I also recognized that I would not have been happy with any facility. Dad was safe and fed and not in any visible emotional distress or pain. Sometimes that is the best you can do.

Like me, many individuals view full-time care facilities, such as nursing homes, as either unnecessary or negative in some way. Due to this misconception, many caregivers and family members feel extreme guilt when a loved one is placed in a long-term care facility. The truth, however, is that your loved one will likely need some form of full-time care if they are facing significant functional declines or medical complications. The checklist below highlights some signs that your loved one might benefit from a long-term care facility.

Checklist: Signs your loved one could benefit from a long-term care facility

Your loved one:

- ☐ Has been injured due to functional declines.
- ☐ Needs daily medical assistance from a professional.
- ☐ Has one or more serious medical conditions.
- ☐ Needs 24-hour care and supervision.
- ☐ Has begun aspirating or choking on their food regularly.
- ☐ Is now bedridden.
- ☐ Is incontinent and/or is using objects other than the toilet for voiding.
- ☐ Has lost the ability to communicate their needs (through speech, hand gestures, or writing).
- ☐ Needs frequent assistance walking or standing.
- ☐ Is no longer safe in their environment.
- ☐ Requires pain management, medical care, and/or hospice care.
- ☐ Has symptoms that are becoming too much for their caregiver to manage.
- ☐ Needs physical assistance with eating.
- ☐ Requires daily management of medications.

The services provided by long-term care facilities vary based on the type of institution. For example, units that specialize in memory care are geared toward individuals with dementia, whereas nursing homes provide a broader spectrum of care. The following checklist discusses some of the services provided by full-time care facilities.

Checklist: Services provided at full-time care facilities

- ☐ Specialized medical care

- ☐ 24-hour-a-day nursing services

- ☐ Assistance taking medications

- ☐ Prescribing new medications

- ☐ Wound care

- ☐ Preventative care and access to immunizations, such as flu and pneumonia vaccines

- ☐ Arrangements with local hospitals in case of a medical emergency

- ☐ Palliative care (Some facilities will provide hospice services, but in many cases you will need to arrange this yourself if they allow it.)

- ☐ Dental care (Some facilities will provide monthly access to a dentist, but this is not the case in all areas so check with the individual facility.)

- ☐ Health and nutrition management

- ☐ Three balanced meals a day, generally served in a dining room; in some facilities, residents can request food to be served in their room

- ☐ Help with any feeding needs

- ☐ Housekeeping

- ☐ Laundry

- ☐ Assistance bathing and dressing

- ☐ Monitoring and assistance with personal hygiene

- ☐ Assistance with toileting and the use of garments for incontinence

- ☐ Recreational activities with other residents

- ☐ Activities and programs to promote physical exercise

- ☐ Memory retention activities

- ☐ Religious and cultural programs and activities

- ☐ Physical therapy and speech therapy

- ☐ A secure environment with 24-hour-a-day monitoring

When deciding on a full-time care facility, you should visit the facility at different parts of the day and week to see how the staff interacts with residents, how activities such as meal times are conducted, and how the environment changes with different staff and activities. For example, visit the facility both in the morning and at meal times to see how much the noise volume increases. You can also go on your state's website to check how the home is rated overall for service and quality. The following checklist highlights some areas to pay particular attention to when deciding on a long-term care facility.

Checklist: Questions to consider when looking for a full-time care facility

- ☐ Do they admit patients with your loved one's specific condition?

- ☐ Do they have a special unit for your loved one's condition? If so, how is it different than the other units?

- ☐ Is the staff trained to work with patients who have your loved one's condition?

- ☐ Will they provide you with a sample care plan for a resident similar to your loved one?

- ☐ Does the facility perform background checks on all employees? What

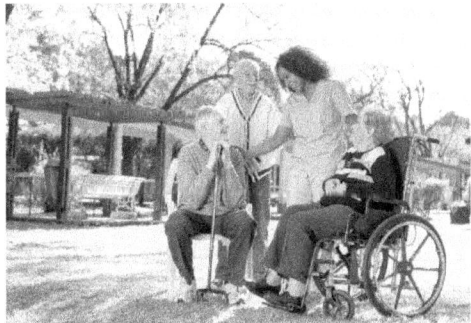

Credit: GaliardiImages

47

are their hiring restrictions in accordance with these background checks? In other words, if a person has ever been suspected of abuse or mistreatment, will the facility still hire them?

- ☐ What is their policy for a staff member who uses physical force against a resident? It should be zero-tolerance.

- ☐ What kind of security is in place if a resident wanders or becomes confused?

- ☐ Where are the cameras at the facility located? Will you be able to have access to the footage if needed (such as in cases of suspected abuse)?

- ☐ Do they have activities available every day?

- ☐ How much social interaction do residents have with staff and one another?

- ☐ Do residents share rooms with one another, or are there single rooms available?

- ☐ Is there an outside area for residents?

- ☐ How are meal times handled?

- ☐ How many people are available to help the resident eat?

- ☐ Can residents eat in their rooms if they wish?

- ☐ How does the staff promote and/or monitor healthy nutrition?

- ☐ What forms of nutritional assessment will be conducted? How often will these assessments be conducted?

- ☐ Are families encouraged to participate in activities, meal times, and overall care?

- ☐ How are medications stored? (They should be locked.)

- ☐ Do the residents at the facility appear to be happy?

- ☐ Are the current residents well-groomed and dressed appropriately?

- [ ] Is the staff friendly and respectful?

- [ ] Is the setup/design of the facility easy to navigate?

- [ ] What are the visiting hours? Do those hours work with your schedule?

- [ ] What is the ratio of nurses and doctors to residents?

- [ ] What is the ratio of social workers to residents?

- [ ] What is the ratio of nurses (RNs) to staff/CNAs to staff on the days and on the weekends?

- [ ] What is the employee turnover rate?

- [ ] What policies are in place in the case of a medical emergency?

- [ ] Do they provide hospice services if they are needed?

- [ ] Can your loved one's living space be decorated in any way they choose?

- [ ] What religious and/or cultural services do they have in place for residents?

- [ ] What doctors will be caring for your loved one, and will you be able to meet and approve them before any care is given?

- [ ] What is the reputation of the facility?

- [ ] Does the facility currently have any citations pending against them? If so, how serious are the citations?

- [ ] Has the facility had citations in the past?

- [ ] Is the facility covered by your loved one's insurance provider?

- [ ] How long is the waiting list to get a bed at the facility? Will it be longer if your loved one is on Medicaid?

- [ ] How will you be billed for services? What extras should you expect on top of the monthly fee (i.e., haircuts, activities, incontinence briefs, gloves)?

- [ ] Can you speak to current staff, residents, and the family members of residents before you choose the facility?

□ Is the facility overly noisy? What is the facility's policy on noise control?

□ What types of activities are offered to residents? How frequently are activities held?

Memory Care Units

Some assisted living and long-term care facilities are specifically tailored to those with Alzheimer's disease and other forms of dementia. They are called memory care units, special care units, or memory support programs. These units are generally set apart from the other areas of the facility and have dedicated staff. Short-term or long-term care facilities that offer these specialized programs can be very beneficial if your loved one has dementia. Your loved one will be around others who have memory difficulties, and the staff will be trained to work with individuals who have dementia. The following checklist details some of the features of memory care units.

Checklist: Features of memory care units

□ All residents have either dementia or Alzheimer's disease.

□ Staff has specialized training to care for those with dementia or Alzheimer's disease.

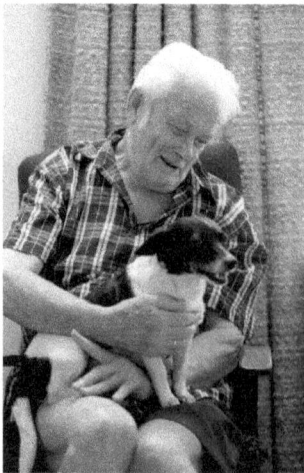

Credit: Nolte Lourens

□ Staff receives frequent training in order to stay knowledgeable about new research, findings, and changes to suggested care practices.

□ Activities and games are aimed at memory retention.

□ Enhanced safety protocols are in place.

□ Large signs and other measures are in place to help decrease disorientation and confusion.

- ☐ Often provide a higher degree of individualized attention.

- ☐ Feature private or semi-private living areas.

- ☐ Rooms are designed to promote resident independence.

- ☐ Both nurses and social workers provide 24-hour supervision and care.

- ☐ The ratio of nurses and doctors to residents to provide specialized and dedicated care is high.

- ☐ More pet, music, art, and relaxation therapies are available.

- ☐ Personalized programs are tailored to help individual residents.

- ☐ A larger emphasis is placed on recreational and social activities to promote stimulation and avoid sedentary activities.

Memory care units are designed specifically for individuals with Alzheimer's disease or other forms of dementia. As such, a facility like this would be an ideal place if your loved one is experiencing these problems and if you can find one in your area that is covered by your loved one's insurance or otherwise affordable.

Psychiatric Facilities

In some cases, individuals with Alzheimer's disease, dementia, and other problems with cognition may develop problems with aggression or violence. If this is the case for your loved one, they may be placed in a psychiatric facility, especially if they were in an assisted living or long-term care facility and injured a caregiver or another resident. Care facilities must protect their workers and residents and having a resident who is a danger to others is a liability many facilities will not tolerate. If you are unable to handle the care of your loved one outside of a long-term care facility, your loved one may be placed in a psychiatric facility and held involuntarily until the situation subsides. To understand more about psychiatric facilities, see the following checklists.

Checklist: Reasons your loved one may be placed in a psychiatric facility

- ☐ Biting

- ☐ Hitting

- ☐ Pushing

- ☐ Cussing

- ☐ Pulling hair

- ☐ Delusions

- ☐ Paranoia

- ☐ Hallucinations

- ☐ Fighting

- ☐ Threatening someone with a sharp object

- ☐ Spitting

- ☐ Mood swings

- ☐ Threatening to commit suicide

- ☐ Yelling

- ☐ Stomping on someone

Checklist: What to expect from a psychiatric facility

- ☐ Your loved one may be held for 72 hours or more without your approval.

- ☐ Your loved one should be assessed by a physician.

- ☐ The physician will likely try different combinations of medications to control aggressive or psychiatric symptoms.

- ☐ The physician will likely try to identify triggers for psychiatric or aggressive behavior. For individuals with cognitive problems, seemingly unlikely triggers can cause aggression, such as a change in environment, asking your loved one to change clothing, or trying to force them to take medication or take a bath.

- ☐ Your loved one may be placed in a solitary room.

- ☐ Your loved one may be restrained by the arms and/or legs.

- ☐ Your loved one's health and mental acuity may decline rapidly after a stay in a psychiatric facility, or it may improve if the physicians find a better combination of medications.

- ☐ Your loved one may need a court order to release them from the psychiatric facility.

- ☐ Your loved one will likely have a harder time finding another long-term care facility to take them after their release from the psychiatric facility.

If your loved one has dementia or is experiencing cognitive problems, you and your family may want to be prepared by choosing a psychiatric facility that you would like your loved one transported to in case of emergency. Once you have made this choice, notify your loved one's assisted living or long-term care facility of your decision and ask them to honor your wishes should your loved one need to be placed in a psychiatric facility. Questions to ask when choosing a psychiatric facility are listed below.

Checklist: Questions to ask when choosing a psychiatric facility

- ☐ What is the physician-to-patient ratio? What is the nurse-to-patient ratio?

- ☐ Are physicians available for consultations and appointments over the weekend and on holidays? Or will your loved one be required to wait over the weekend or holiday before being assessed?

- ☐ Do the physicians, nurses, and other employees have experience dealing with behaviors of individuals with your loved one's condition?

- ☐ Do the physicians have experience successfully finding medication combinations that can control behavioral changes in your loved one without making them lethargic?

- ☐ Does the facility have a standard protocol for dealing with acts of aggression? If so, what is it? Is it something you are comfortable with?

- ☐ What is the facility's policy on solitary confinement?

- ☐ What is the facility's policy on restraints?

- ☐ Does the facility have a history of reported abuse?

- ☐ Does the facility provide opportunities for mental stimulation and physical activity?

- ☐ Will the facility help your loved one with activities of daily living (e.g., bathing, eating, toileting) if your loved one is unable to do this on their own?

- ☐ Will you be allowed to visit your loved one in the psychiatric facility? If so, what are the visiting hours?

- ☐ What is the overall environment of the psychiatric facility? Does it provide a calm atmosphere? Are residents too isolated?

- ☐ What fees are associated with a voluntary vs. involuntary stay at the psychiatric facility?

- ☐ Will the facility accept your loved one's healthcare or long-term care insurance?

- ☐ How close is the psychiatric facility to your house and your loved one's care facility?

- ☐ What is the facility's policy about releasing your loved one into your care if they were placed in the psychiatric facility by your loved one's assisted living or long-term care facility?

Although having your loved one committed to a psychiatric facility is difficult emotionally, knowing what to expect and being prepared for this possibility will make the transition easier for you. Having a plan in place that your family, your loved one, and your loved one's care facility agree on will make the transition much smoother, and it will prevent any surprises that would cause undue emotional stress.

Elder Abuse in Care Facilities

Elder abuse and neglect are important concerns for older adults who depend on someone else for care. In 2017, an estimated 1 in 6 older adults experienced elder abuse. The risk of abuse is greatest for those who are frail, have a disability, or have Alzheimer's disease or other forms of dementia.

There are several common types of elder abuse. The first is physical abuse, which includes hitting, pushing, and any other action that causes physical harm. The second type is emotional abuse, in which psychological harm is inflicted through words or actions. It involves yelling, threatening, and intimidating. Preventing contact between an older adult and their friends or family is a form of emotional abuse.

A third type of abuse is sexual abuse. It involves forcing an older adult to participate in or watch sexual acts. Fourth is neglect, which is the failure to fulfill caretaking duties. The caregiver's lack of response to the older adult's needs may be intentional or unintentional.

Finally, financial abuse is unauthorized use of financial assets. It may include theft of property, misuse of financial instruments, and identity theft or forgery.

Cognitive problems make it difficult for an individual to recognize and report abuse. It can also make the individual a target for would-be abusers. Abusers may be family

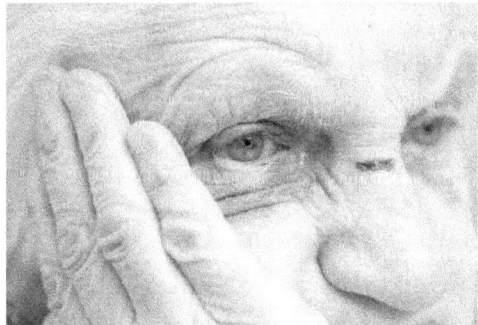

Credit: Ocskay Mark

members, caregivers, healthcare providers, and employees of or other residents at a care facility. When spending time with your loved one, you must be observant for signs of abuse or neglect. The following checklist includes questions that may help you determine if your loved has experienced abuse. When considering these questions, note that some signs of elder abuse mimic symptoms of other age-related medical conditions.

Checklist: Signs of elder abuse

☐ Does your loved one have unexplained injuries (bruises, burns, or scars)?

☐ Has your loved one developed pressure ulcers or other preventable problems?

☐ Does your loved one look messy? Is their hair unwashed or their clothes dirty?

☐ Has your loved one lost weight for no reason?

☐ Does your loved one have trouble sleeping?

☐ Is your loved one depressed?

☐ Does your loved one display signs of trauma (such as rocking back and forth)?

☐ Is your loved one uncharacteristically agitated or violent?

☐ Has your loved one withdrawn from others or activities they previously enjoyed?

☐ Does your loved one often request to leave the facility?

When signs suggest your loved one has been abused, do your best to gather information. Initially, try talking with your loved one. Your ability to gather information this way may be limited if your loved one has experienced declines in cognitive functioning or communication skills. Frame your conversation and questions in a way that suggests an interest in how they are feeling and what they have been doing since you last visited.

If your loved one is capable of answering your questions but seems reluctant to do so, make sure you are in a private location. Older adults who have been abused may fear reprisals from their abuser if they confide in others. Their reluctance to speak up may come from a fear of being overheard.

Observe interactions between your loved one and others, if possible. This includes facility staff and other residents. Note any changes in your loved one's behavior or personality when others are in the room. Observe their body language as well. If your loved one pulls away from the other person or moves closer to you, this may indicate a problem. Their voice may also drop in pitch or volume, or they may stop talking altogether.

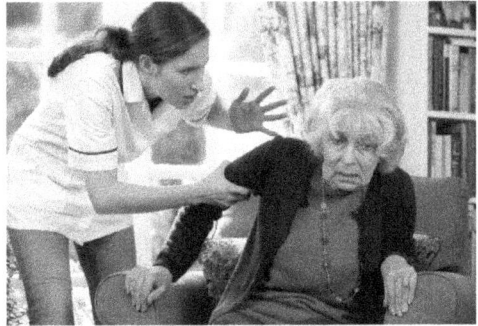
Credit: SpeedKingz

Other indicators of abuse include staff preventing you from seeing or speaking to your loved one during normal hours without a valid reason. Staff members may also refuse to allow you to visit privately with your loved one.

If you believe your loved one has been abused or your loved one accuses someone of abuse, you should report it immediately. This will prevent further suffering by your loved one and, potentially, prevent others in your loved one's facility from being harmed. The following list outlines the type of information that should be included in your report. Additionally, if you feel the danger to your loved one is immediate and life-threatening, call 911.

Checklist: Making a report of elder abuse

- ☐ Make your report in writing and keep a copy of it for your records.

☐ Provide information about who was involved. This includes the name and address of your loved one, as well as the name of the facility in which your loved one lives. The individuals who provide care to your loved one should be named, and the individual you believe abused your loved one should be identified specifically.

☐ Provide information about what happened. This includes the nature and extent of the harm done, as well as any physical signs of abuse. Any previous incidents should also be noted, as well as a description of what occurred (provided that you or someone else witnessed the incident or that your loved one is able to relay that information to you).

☐ Include photographs of any physical injuries. Make sure to seek your loved one's permission for doing so before taking the photographs.

☐ Provide information about where and when. This includes the time, place, and date of the incident, if that can be determined. If you cannot identify the exact day, narrow it down to a timeframe. For example, if you your loved one has a bruise on their face on Friday that was not there on Wednesday, you know the injury took place sometime between Wednesday and Friday.

☐ Sign and date your report.

Remember, the suspicion of abuse is sufficient for making a report. It is not your responsibility to prove that abuse actually occurred—it is the responsibility of the agencies to whom you submit your report. Those agencies may include, but are not limited to, those listed here.

Checklist: Agencies for reporting elder abuse

☐ The facility's administrator, director of nursing, and social worker

☐ The state agency that licenses and certifies nursing homes and investigates complaints; this is often the State Health Department

- Local police or state law enforcement

- A protection and advocacy agency or an adult protective services agency

- The Long-Term Care Ombudsman Program or a similar group that advocates for residents in long-term care facilities

After making your report, regularly follow up with the facility and your loved one to see that the abuse has stopped. Also, follow up with the persons or agencies conducting investigations and ask for copies of their findings, if they are allowed by law to release them.

You may also want to follow up with the licensing agency authorities in your state to make sure they are aware of any charges against the abuser. If accusations of abuse against a nurse aide or licensed staff person are substantiated by a state agency or if a finding of guilt is returned by a court of law, the individual must be reported to the appropriate registry or licensing board. Facilities must not engage individuals with these findings as either employees or volunteers. They may also not engage individuals who have had disciplinary action taken against a professional license.

The Moving Process

Moving to a new place can be hard on your loved one, no matter their physical or mental state, or if they are moving out of choice or necessity. Major moves should be planned long ahead of the move, if possible, in order to ensure the best acclimation to the new environment. When your loved one's surroundings change, this will likely cause a great deal of stress, even if the move goes perfectly. If your loved one does become stressed, they may exhibit difficult behaviors or become

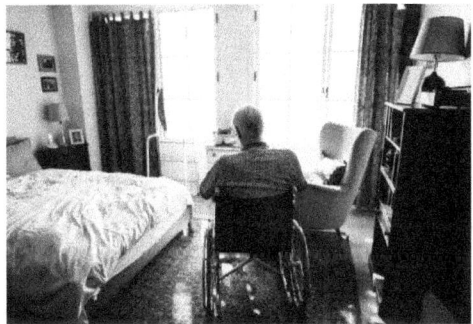

Credit: Rawpixel.com

withdrawn. Both reactions are entirely normal, as long as they begin to subside in a reasonable amount of time. Keep in mind that acclimating to a new environment does not occur overnight. Sometimes it could take your loved one two to three weeks to become comfortable with their new living environment. Depending on your loved one's reaction to the move, you and other family members may have to avoid visiting for a time to allow your loved one to get used to the new surroundings. In addition, a number of steps can be taken to ensure that the move and subsequent transition are as smooth as possible.

Checklist: Easing the transition

- ☐ Bring your loved one to the facility a few times before they move in.

- ☐ Talk to the staff about your loved one's habits, favorite foods, preferred activities, etc.

- ☐ Inform the staff about any daily rituals or schedules your loved one generally follows.

- ☐ Decorate your loved one's room before the move-in day.

- ☐ Bring familiar pictures, blankets, quilts, and decorations for your loved one's new room.

- ☐ If your loved one has a favorite chair or piece of furniture, consider bringing it for their room.

- ☐ Put together scrap books or photo albums with pictures of loved ones, and label the pictures with names.

- ☐ Decorate the walls with family photos.

- ☐ Move items from your loved one's old home to the new residence when your loved one is not around.

- ☐ Be positive during the move and when talking to your loved one about the new place.

- ☐ Have at least two people at the facility when your loved one moves in; this way, one person can fill out any paperwork and talk to the staff while the other person stays with your loved one.

☐ When you leave, try not to make a big production; instead, slip away quietly.

☐ Recognize that it will take a few weeks for your loved one to become acclimated to the new surroundings.

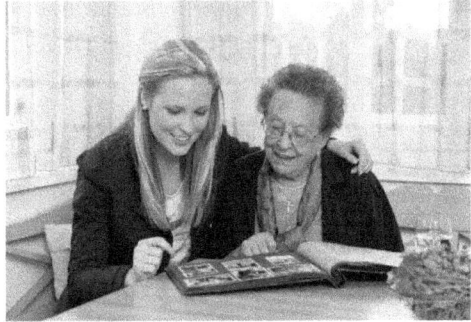

☐ If your loved one becomes agitated or stressed when you visit in the first few weeks, consider limiting your visits in order to ease their transition.

Credit: Lisa S.

Conclusion

Many options exist for living arrangements. If your loved one enjoys good physical and mental health, they may be able to stay home and maintain their independence; as they age or their health changes, they may need to move in with a caregiver or move to an assisted living or long-term care facility. These decisions are not easy to make, which is why you and your loved should discuss their preferences early in the aging process while they are in good health. If you and your family have never had to organize care for a loved one who was ill, the process can be difficult to navigate. Knowing what questions to ask and what features to look for in care facilities can be tremendously valuable. This process is not something you have to go through alone, and there are numerous resources available that can help you organize care for your loved one. Caring for an elderly loved one with physical or cognitive problems does not only affect the individual, it impacts the family of that individual as well.

About the Authors

Laura Town

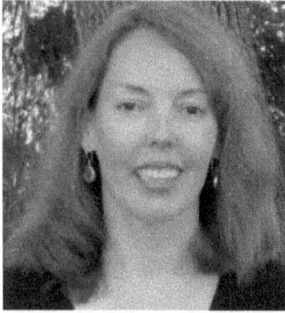

Laura Town has authored numerous publications of special interest to the aging population. She has expertise in the field of finance as a co-author on *Finance: Foundations of Financial Institutions and Management* published by John Wiley and Sons, and she has contributed to several online nursing courses and texts. She has also written for the American Medical Writers Association, and her work has been published by the American Society of Journalists and Authors. As an editor, Laura has worked with Pearson Education, Prentice Hall, McGraw-Hill Higher Education, John Wiley and Sons, and the University of Pennsylvania to create both on-ground and online courses and texts. She has previously served as the President of the Indiana chapter of the American Medical Writers Association.

Karen (Kassel) Hoffman

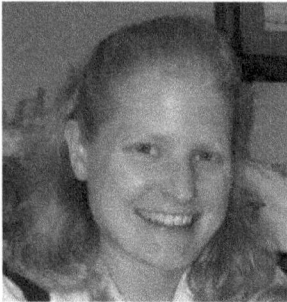

Karen (Kassel) Hoffman received her Ph.D. in Pharmacology from the Department of Pharmacology and Experimental Neurosciences at the University of Nebraska Medical Center in Omaha, NE, where she was the recipient of an American Heart Association fellowship and several regional and national awards for her research on G protein-coupled receptor signaling in airways. She then pursued post-doctoral research projects at the University of North Carolina-Chapel Hill and the University of Kansas Medical Center, again receiving fellowships from the PhRMA Foundation and the American Heart Association, respectively. She has published research in the *American Journal of Pathology*, *Journal of Biological Chemistry*, and *Journal of Pharmacology and Experimental Therapeutics*. In 2012, Karen joined the editorial staff at

WilliamsTown Communications, an editing firm that specializes in educational products for undergraduate- and graduate-level students. At WTC, Karen specializes in producing educational products related to the sciences and healthcare. In addition, Karen is board-certified for editing life sciences (BELS-certified).

A Note from the Authors

Thank you for purchasing our book! Worldwide, roughly 617 million people are aged 65 and over, and that number is expected to increase to 1.6 billion by 2050. In the United States, approximately 47 million people currently fall into this age group.

People today are living longer, but that does not necessarily mean they are living better. Odds are good that your loved one will be affected by one or more health conditions. Noncommunicable diseases are a major health concern among people age 60 and older in the United States. These include conditions like heart disease (43 million people affected), diabetes (12 million), and Alzheimer's disease (5 million). Despite the fact that many older adults—and their caregivers—face these health concerns, you may feel alone. I (Laura) know that when I started caring for my father, who had early-onset Alzheimer's disease, I felt alone. Although my father has passed away, I am haunted by what he suffered and how difficult it was to care for him. However, now I know that there are people, resources, and organizations that can help others going through this or similar struggles.

No matter the condition their loved one faces, caregivers have emotional, physical, and financial challenges. We hope that the information in this book will ease some of your stress. The steps included here can help you recognize the signs that a new living situation is needed, as well as aid you in assessing that living situation for safety and quality. All of the steps may not apply to every situation, but they will stimulate your thinking and get you progressing forward in the moving process. In addition, we have included resources at the end of this book to provide additional information to help you through this process.

If you have any questions for us, feel free to post them on Laura Town's Amazon Author Central page or reach out to her via twitter: @laurawtown. **We would appreciate it if you would take the time to review our book on Amazon, as our book's visibility on Amazon depends on reviews.**

Additional Titles from Omega Press

Alzheimer's Roadmap series:

Long-Term Care Insurance, Power of Attorney, Wealth Management, and Other First Steps

Dementia, Alzheimer's Disease Stages, Treatment Options, and Other Medical Considerations

Advance Directives, Durable Power of Attorney, Wills, and Other Legal Considerations

Home Safety Checklist Guide and Caregiver Resources for Medication Safety, Driving, and Wandering

Caregiver Resources: From Independence to a Memory Care Unit

Caregiver Resources for Helping with Activities of Daily Living

Nutrition for Brain Health: Fighting Dementia

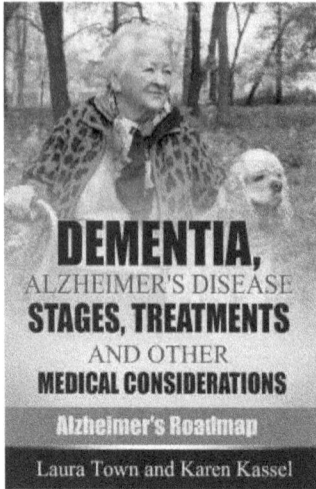

A guide to Alzheimer's disease progression and treatment

Dementia, Alzheimer's Disease Stages, Treatments, and Other Medical Considerations provides answers to the following questions and more:

- **What is Alzheimer's disease?** This book describes what Alzheimer's disease is, including its characteristics, warning signs, and risk factors.
- **What can my loved one with Alzheimer's disease expect?** Read detailed descriptions of the general stages of Alzheimer's disease, including what patients and caregivers can expect to see at each stage as the disease progresses.
- **What treatments are available?** A survey of prescription medications introduces you to the treatments available to help patients with Alzheimer's disease cope with the progression of the disease. Also find out which drugs to *avoid*. An additional review of alternative treatments assesses the efficacy and veracity of some of these treatments.

> *"Best resource I have found for explaining in terms I can understand about what my husband is experiencing and will be going through."*
>
> Kindle Customer

- **What about clinical trials?** Clinical trials are important to finding a cure for Alzheimer's disease, but this book describes the precautions your loved one to consider before choosing to participate in them.
- **Is there audio for this book?** Yes, you can find the audiobook here: https://adbl.co/2SwzzlA

Simple dietary changes can improve cognition and decrease dementia risk and progression

NUTRITION FOR BRAIN HEALTH
Fighting Dementia

Alzheimer's Roadmap

Laura Town, Karen Kassel, and Amanda Boyle

Nutrition for Brain Health: Fighting Dementia provides answers to the following questions and more:

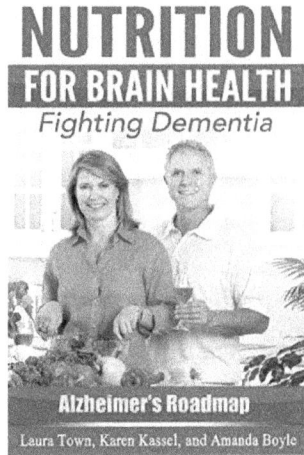

- **How can what I eat affect my brain health?** Discover how to lower you risk factors for dementia by decreasing your intake of saturated fats and cholesterol, balancing your diet, and controlling the calories you consume.
- **Do I need to exercise?** Explore the various ways that everyday activities can double as brain-enhancing exercise and improve your total health as well.
- **Does what I drink matter?** Find out how some things you may drink, such as coffee, tea, or red wine, can actually be beneficial for brain health in moderation.
- **How do I get the vitamins I need?** Know what dietary and lifestyle choices can increase your intake of essential vitamins such as vitamins C and B_{12}.
- **How do I know what specific foods are good for me?** This book defines the elements of a healthy, balanced diet and then goes beyond that to identify the specific foods that will give you the nutrients you need to extend and improve cognitive function.
- **Is there an electronic version of this book?** Yes, and it's free!
- **Is there an audio version of this book?** Yes, there is. You can find it at: https://adbl.co/2Vwbe0d

Resources

Caring Bridge

Website: http://www.caringbridge.org/

This website will help you to coordinate caregiving help with family and friends.

Eldercare Locator

Phone: 1-800-272-3900

Website: http://www.eldercare.acl.gov/Public/index.aspx

This website will help you to find long and short-term care facilities in your area.

National Care Planning Council

Website: http://www.longtermcarelink.net/a7nursinghome.htm

This website has links to care providers, services, and advisors broken down by state.

Nursing Home Compare

Website: http://www.medicare.gov/nursinghomecompare/search.html

This website provides information about every nursing home in the country that is Medicare or Medicaid certified.

Senior Living

Website: http://www.seniorliving.org/lifestyles/memory-care/

This website provides a list of long-term and short-term care facilities in your area, as well as resources for local homecare services.

Meals on Wheels America

1550 Crystal Drive, Suite 1004

Arlington, VA 22202

Phone: 888-998-6325

Fax: 703-548-5274

Email: info@mealsonwheelsamerica.org

Website: http://www.mealsonwheelsamerica.org/

Website to find a Meals on Wheels in your area:

http://www.mealsonwheelsamerica.org/signup/aboutmealsonwheels/find-programs

Caregiver Agreement Example

Maine: http://www.maine.gov/dhhs/ofi/documents/LTC-Personal-Support-Agreement.pdf

Reference List

Administration for Community Living. (2018). Home health care. Retrieved from https://www.acl.gov/sites/default/files/news%202017-03/Home_Health_Care.pdf.

Aging Life Care Association. (2018). What you need to know. Retrieved from www.aginglifecare.org/ALCA/About_Aging_Life_Care/What_you_need_to_know/ALCA/About_Aging_Life_Care/What_you_need_to_know.aspx?hkey=e3b15907-97b1-4a4a-acac-cc1d515bd311.

Alzheimer's Association. (2018). Alzheimer's disease facts and figures. Retrieved from https://www.alz.org/documents_custom/2018-facts-and-figures.pdf.

American Association of Retired Persons (AARP). (2017). 7 tips for avoiding caregiver burnout that really work. Retrieved from https://www.aarp.org/caregiving/life-balance/info-2017/avoid-caregiver-fatigue-fd.html.

American Association of Retired Persons (AARP) Public Policy Institute. (2010). Fact sheet: Home modifications to promote independent living. Retrieved from https://www.aarp.org/content/dam/aarp/livable-communities/learn/housing/home-modifications-to-promote-independent-living-2010-aarp.pdf.

American Diabetes Association. (2018). Overall numbers, diabetes and prediabetes. Retrieved from www.diabetes.org/diabetes-basics/statistics/.

American Heart Association. (2016). Older Americans & cardiovascular diseases. Retrieved from https://www.heart.org/idc/groups/heart-public/@wcm/@sop/@smd/documents/downloadable/ucm_4839 70.pdf.

Argentum. (2017). Guide to choosing a senior living community. Retrieved from https://www.argentum.org/wp-content/uploads/2017/08/Argentum-Guide-to-Choosing-a-Senior-Living-Community.pdf.

Blue Apron. (2017). Help center. Retrieved from https://support.blueapron.com/hc/en-us/categories/115000487547-Meals.

Centers for Medicare & Medicaid Services. (2017). Your guide to choosing a nursing home or other long-term care. Retrieved from https://www.medicare.gov/Pubs/pdf/02174-Nursing-Home-Other-Long-Term-Services.pdf.

Economics and Statistics Administration. (2017). Older Americans month: May 2017. Retrieved from https://www.census.gov/content/dam/Census/newsroom/facts-for-features/2017/cb17-ff08.pdf.

Family Caregiver Alliance. (2017). Personal care agreements: How to compensate a family member for providing care. Retrieved from https://caregiver.org/personal-care-agreements.

Federal Interagency Forum on Aging-Related Statistics. (2016). Older Americans: Key indicators of well-being. Retrieved from https://agingstats.gov/docs/LatestReport/Older-Americans-2016-Key-Indicators-of-WellBeing.pdf.

Fisher Center for Alzheimer's Research Foundation. (2018). Assisted living facilities. Retrieved from http://www.alzinfo.org/08/treatment-care/assisted-living-facilities.

Fisher Center for Alzheimer's Research Foundation. (2018). Stop elder abuse. Retrieved from https://www.alzinfo.org/articles/stop-elder-abuse/.

Gross, J. (2008, October 6). Why hire a Geriatric Care Manager? *The New York Times*. Retrieved from http://newoldage.blogs.nytimes.com/2008/10/06/why-hire-a-geriatric-care-manager/?_php=true&_type=blogs&_php=true&_type=blogs&_php=true&_type=blogs&_php=true&_type=blogs&_r=3&.

Helpguide.org. (2018). Elder abuse and neglect: Spotting the warning signs and getting help. Retrieved from https://www.helpguide.org/articles/abuse/elder-abuse-and-neglect.htm.

Leonhardt, M. (2017, July 19). This is the best meal-kit service on the market right now. *Money*. Retrieved from http://time.com/money/4856342/best-meal-kits-value/.

National Consumer Voice for Quality Long-Term Care. (2017). Fact sheet: Abuse, neglect, exploitation, and misappropriation of property. Retrieved from http://theconsumervoice.org/uploads/files/long-term-care-recipient/abuse-fact-sheet-18.pdf.

National Institute on Aging. (2016). Elder abuse. Retrieved from https://www.nia.nih.gov/health/elder-abuse#signs.

National Institute on Aging. (2017). Getting help with Alzheimer's caregiving. Retrieved from https://www.nia.nih.gov/health/getting-help-alzheimers-caregiving.

National Institute on Aging. (2017). Alzheimer's caregiving: Caring for yourself. Retrieved from https://www.nia.nih.gov/health/alzheimers-caregiving-caring-yourself.

National Institutes of Health. (2016). World's older population grows dramatically. Retrieved from https://www.nih.gov/news-events/news-releases/worlds-older-population-grows-dramatically.

Peck, K. (2016). Creating effective agreements for payment of family caregivers. *Bifocal* 37 (3): 63–65. Retrieved from https://www.americanbar.org/publications/bifocal/vol_37/issue_3_february2016/creating-effective-caregiver-agreements.html.

Shipt. (2018). How can we help? Retrieved from https://help.shipt.com/.

World Health Organization (WHO). (2018). Elder abuse. Retrieved from www.who.int/en/news-room/fact-sheets/detail/elder-abuse.

www.ingramcontent.com/pod-product-compliance
Lightning Source LLC
Chambersburg PA
CBHW032119280326
41933CB00009B/916